Implementing
Group and Individual
Medical
Nutrition Therapy
for Diabetes

Marion J. Franz, MS, RD, CDE
Diane Reader, RD, CDE
Arlene Monk, RD, CDE

▲. American Diabetes Association.
Cure • Care • Commitment℠

Director, Book Publishing, John Fedor; *Associate Director, Professional Books*, Christine B. Welch; *Editor*, Joyce Raynor; *Production Manager*, Peggy M. Rote; *Composition*, Circle Graphics, Inc.; *Cover Design*, Koncept, Inc.; *Printer*, Graphic Communications, Inc.

Printed in the United States of America
1 3 5 7 9 10 8 6 4 2

ADA titles may be purchased for business or promotional use or for special sales. To purchase this book in large quantities, or for custom editions with your logo, contact Lee Romano Sequeira, Special Sales & Promotions, at the address below, or at LRomano@diabetes.org, or call 703-299-2046.

American Diabetes Association
1701 North Beauregard Street
Alexandria, Virginia 22311

Library of Congress Cataloging-in-Publication Data

Franz, Marion J.
    Implementing group and individual medical nutrition therapy for diabetes / Marion J. Franz, Diane Reader, Arlene Monk.
        p. ; cm.
    Includes bibliographical references and index.
    ISBN 1-58040-165-1 (pbk. : alk. paper)
        1. Diabetes–Diet therapy. 2. Patient education. I. Reader, Diane. II. Monk, Arlene. III. Title.
        [DNLM: 1. Diabetes Mellitus–diet therapy. 2. Diet Therapy–methods. WK 818 F837i 2002] RC662 .F7365 2002
    616.4'620654–dc21

                                                                                    2002066717

Contents

Acknowledgments

The material in this book is a synthesis of the processes used for providing medical nutrition therapy for individuals with diabetes over the past 20 plus years at the International Diabetes Center in Minneapolis. We are indebted to our colleagues for their support and to the many patients who have been our best teachers during this time. The process has been implemented, evaluated, and implemented and evaluated again and again. It has been presented in an uncountable number of lectures in *Team Management of Diabetes* at the International Diabetes Center. It is a process that is always changing as we continue to learn how to better facilitate lifestyle changes. Our goal as authors is to help readers and other professionals better implement effective medical nutrition therapy.

Implementing
Group and **Individual**
Medical
Nutrition Therapy
for Diabetes

1

Guidelines for Medical Nutrition Therapy for Diabetes

Managing diabetes is a team effort. Dietitians, nurses, physicians, behavioral counselors, and other health care providers contribute their expertise to the development of therapeutic regimens that assist individuals with diabetes to achieve the best possible metabolic control. People with diabetes must be at the center of the team because they have the responsibility of day-to-day implementation of management. The goal of medical nutrition therapy (MNT) is to provide individuals with the knowledge, skills, and motivation to incorporate lifestyle self-management into their daily lives.

In this chapter, you will find a summary of nutrition guidelines. Professionals can use these guidelines to provide current and accurate knowledge and skills to individuals with diabetes. Nutrition principles and recommendations were updated in 2002 and are now classified according to the level of supporting scientific evidence (1,2). Motivating or assisting individuals with diabetes to make lifestyle changes is discussed in Chapter 2. Chapters 3 and 4 review the process for providing the knowledge and skills for making appropriate food choices and increasing physical activity to people with diabetes either in groups or individually. The Appendix includes sample forms and figures that the reader may find useful.

Goals of Medical Nutrition Therapy (1,2)

1. To attain and maintain optimal metabolic outcomes, including
   - blood glucose levels in the normal range or as close to normal as is safely possible
   - a lipid and lipoprotein profile that reduces the risk for cardiovascular disease
   - blood pressure levels that reduce risk for vascular disease
2. To prevent or treat the chronic complications of diabetes—dyslipidemia, hypertension, cardiovascular disease, nephropathy, neuropathy
3. To improve health through healthful food choices and physical activity
4. To address individual needs—personal and cultural preferences and lifestyle—taking into account the individual's wishes, willingness, and ability to change

Effectiveness of Medical Nutrition Therapy

Research supports MNT as an effective therapy in reaching treatment goals for glycemia, lipids, and blood pressure. Outcomes studies demonstrated that MNT provided by registered dietitians was associated with an ~1% decrease in hemoglobin A1C (A1C) in patients with newly diagnosed type 1 diabetes (3), ~2% decrease in A1C in patients with newly diagnosed type 2 diabetes (4,5), and ~1% decrease in A1C in patients with an average 4-year duration of type 2 diabetes (5). All of these improvements occurred without changes in medication and are similar to those from oral glucose-lowering medications. By 6 weeks to 3 months, it was known whether nutrition interventions had led to target blood glucose goals; if not, the dietitian made recommendations to the referral source that changes be made in medications. In a cross-sectional survey examining the role of nutrition behaviors in achieving improved glycemic control in 623 intensively treated patients in the Diabetes Control and Complications Trial, those who reported adhering to their meal plan >90% of the time had 0.9% lower A1C than those who reported adhering to their meal plan <45% of the time (6).

In a meta-analysis of nondiabetic free-living subjects, MNT that restricted saturated fats to 7–10% of energy intake and dietary cholesterol to 200–300 mg/dl daily resulted in a 10–13% (24–32 mg/dl) decrease in total cholesterol, 12–16% (18–25 mg/dl) decrease in LDL cholesterol, and 8% (15–17 mg/dl) decrease in triglycerides (7). HDL cholesterol decreased by 7% with the greater saturated fat restriction; however, adding exercise prevented this decrease.

In a meta-analysis of nondiabetic subjects, moderate reductions in dietary sodium intake (≤2400 mg) decreased blood pressure by 5 mmHg systolic and 2 mmHg diastolic in hypertensive patients and by 3 mmHg systolic and 1 mmHg diastolic in normotensive patients (8). Responses to sodium reduction may be greater in subjects who are "salt sensitive," a characteristic of many patients with diabetes. Clinical trial data suggest that a weight loss of 4.5 kg (10 lb) can be as effective as first-level drugs in controlling blood pressure (9). A low-fat diet that includes fruits and vegetables and low-fat dairy products also reduces blood pressure (10).

Table 1 summarizes the effectiveness of nutrition interventions on metabolic outcomes. Monitor the effect of MNT on glycemic and lipid outcomes approximately 3 months after the initial intervention. Monitor blood pressure at every clinical visit. Table 2 provides key nutrition principles.

TABLE 1: Effectiveness of Medical Nutrition Therapy

Glycemic control	■ 1–2% decrease in A1C ■ 50–100 mg/dl decrease in fasting plasma glucose
Lipids	■ 10–13% decrease in total cholesterol (24–32 mg/dl) ■ 12–16% decrease in LDL cholesterol (18–25 mg/dl) ■ 8% decrease in triglycerides (15–17 mg/dl) ■ Without exercise, HDL cholesterol decreased by 7%; with exercise, no decrease
Hypertension	■ 5-mmHg decrease in systolic blood pressure and 2-mmHg decrease in diastolic blood pressure in hypertensive patients

TABLE 2: Key Nutrition Principles

Nutrition Principles for Type 1 Diabetes (2)	
MNT objectives	■ Develop a food plan based on assessment of an individual's appetite, preferred foods, and usual eating and exercise habits to achieve the goals of MNT. ■ Discuss the food plan with the health care team so that insulin therapy can be integrated into the individual's preferred food/eating and physical activity patterns.

Macronutrients	■ Percentage of macronutrients is based on assessment, metabolic profile, and treatment goals.
	■ The total carbohydrate content of meals (and snacks) is the first priority for food/meal planning and determines post-prandial glucose response and premeal insulin dosage.
	  ● For individuals receiving flexible (intensive) insulin therapy, premeal insulin doses are based on the total amount of carbohydrate in the meal.
	  ● For individuals receiving fixed insulin doses, consistency in day-to-day meal carbohydrate is important.
	■ To avoid weight gain, protein and fat content (energy intake) of the food plan must also be considered.

Exercise	■ For unplanned exercise, additional carbohydrate may be needed. Moderate-intensity exercise increases glucose uptake by ~10–15 g/h. ■ For planned exercise, reduction in insulin dosage may be preferred.
Acute complications	Hypoglycemia ■ Glucose is the preferred treatment for hypoglycemia, although any form of carbohydrate that contains glucose can be used. ■ 15–20 g glucose is an effective but temporary treatment for hypoglycemia. An initial response should be seen in ~10–20 min; however, blood glucose should be evaluated again in ~60 min, as additional treatment may be necessary. Short-term illness ■ During acute illnesses, individuals should continue taking their insulin. ■ Monitor blood glucose and blood or urine for ketones. Drinking adequate amounts of fluids and ingesting carbohydrate are also important during acute illnesses. Oral ingestion of ~150–200 g carbohydrate daily (45–60 g or 3–4 carbohydrate choices every 3–4 h) will reduce or prevent starvation ketosis.

Nutrition Principles for Type 1 Diabetes (2) (*continued*)

Behavioral outcomes	The person with diabetes is able to: ■ Use a food planning system ■ Eat meals/snacks at appropriate times ■ Use information from Nutrition Facts on food labels to determine carbohydrate servings ■ Accurately monitor, record, and use blood glucose data ■ Accurately implement insulin therapy ■ Participate in physical activity per exercise recommendations

Nutrition Principles for Type 2 Diabetes (2)

MNT objectives	■ Implement lifestyle strategies (food plan and physical activity) that will improve clinical outcomes (glycemia, dyslipidemia, and blood pressure). ■ Integrate pharmacological therapy, if needed, into the individual's lifestyle. ■ Use pre- and postmeal blood glucose and A1C tests to determine whether adjustments in food/meal planning will be helpful or medication(s) need to be combined with nutrition therapy.
Macronutrients	■ Percentage of carbohydrate is based on assessment and pre- and postmeal blood glucose data. ■ Teach what foods contain carbohydrate (starches, fruits, starchy vegetables, milk, and sweets), 15-g portion sizes, and the number of servings to select for meals and, if desired, for snacks. ■ Protein and fat content (energy intake) of the food plan also must be considered.
Energy balance and obesity	■ In insulin-resistant individuals, reduced energy intake and modest weight loss improves insulin resistance and glycemia in the short term. Evidence supporting whether this continues long term is not available. ■ Structured, intensive programs that emphasize lifestyle changes, including education, reduced fat and energy intake, regular physical activity, and regular patient contact, are necessary to produce longer-term weight loss on the order of 5–7% of starting weight. ■ Physical activity (exercise) and behavior modification are most useful as adjuncts to other weight loss strategies. Physical activity is important in maintaining weight loss. ■ Reduced-fat diets when maintained long-term contribute to modest loss of weight and improvements in dyslipidemia. ■ Available weight loss drugs should be used only in people with BMI >27 kg/m^2 and in conjunction with lifestyle programs.

(Table 2 continued)

TABLE 2: Key Nutrition Principles (*continued*)

Nutrition Principles for Type 2 Diabetes (2)

	■ Gastric reduction surgery should only be considered in people with BMI >35 kg/m².
Physical activity	■ Physical activity improves insulin sensitivity, glycemia, and lipids; reduces risk for cardiovascular disease; and is helpful in maintenance of weight loss. ■ A minimum cumulative total of 1000 kcal/week from physical activities is recommended (walking 1 mile = ~100 kcal).
Spacing of meals	■ Food frequency, 3 meals or smaller meals and snacks, is based on individual preferences and/or insulin regimen. ■ When insulin is required, consistency in timing of meals and carbohydrate content is important.
Behavioral outcomes	The person with diabetes is able to: ■ Eat meals/snacks at appropriate times ■ Choose food and amounts per food plan ■ Accurately use Nutrition Facts on food labels ■ Participate in physical activity per exercise prescription ■ Appropriately follow prescribed medication regimen ■ Discuss blood glucose monitoring data with health care team or, based on data, make therapy changes as instructed

Nutrient Recommendations for Type 1 and Type 2 Diabetes (1,2)

Carbohydrate	■ Foods containing carbohydrate from whole grains, fruits, vegetables, and low-fat milk are important components of a healthy diet. ■ The total amount of carbohydrate in meals and snacks is more important than the source (starch or sugar) or type (glycemic index). ■ Carbohydrate and monounsaturated fat together should provide 60–70% of energy intake. However, consider the need for weight loss when determining the monounsaturated fat content of the diet.
Sweeteners	■ Sucrose and sucrose-containing foods do not need to be restricted; however, they should be substituted for other carbohydrate sources or, if added, covered with insulin or other glucose-lowering medication(s), and should be eaten within the context of a healthy diet. ■ Nonnutritive sweeteners are safe when consumed within the acceptable daily intake (ADI) levels established by the Food and Drug Administration.

Nutrient Recommendations for Type 1 and Type 2 Diabetes (1,2) (*continued*)

Glycemic index and fiber	■ The use of low–glycemic index foods may reduce postprandial hyperglycemia, but long-term benefits are unclear. ■ Consumption of fiber is encouraged, but there is no reason to recommend that people with diabetes consume more than that recommended for other Americans. Although large amounts (~50 g/day) may have beneficial effects, it is not known whether such high levels of fiber intake can be maintained long term.

Protein	■ In individuals with controlled diabetes, ingested protein does not increase blood glucose levels but is as potent a stimulant of insulin secretion as carbohydrate.
	■ Usual protein intake (15–20% of total daily energy) does not need to be modified if renal function is normal.
	■ Contrary to advice often given, available evidence suggests that:
	  ● Protein does not slow the absorption of carbohydrate.
	  ● Protein combined with carbohydrate does not raise glucose level later than carbohydrate alone and thus does not prevent late-onset hypoglycemia.
	  ● Adding protein to carbohydrate does not assist in the treatment of hypoglycemia or prevent subsequent hypoglycemia.

Dietary fat	■ <10% of energy intake should come from saturated fats; individuals with LDL cholesterol >100 mg/dl may benefit from lowering saturated fats to <7%. ■ Saturated fat can be reduced if weight loss is desirable or replaced with either carbohydrate or monounsaturated fats if weight loss is not the goal. ■ Dietary cholesterol should be <300 mg/dl; individuals with LDL cholesterol >100 mg/dl may benefit from lowering cholesterol to <200 mg/dl. ■ Intake of trans fatty acids should be minimized. ■ ~10% of total energy intake should come from polyunsaturated fatty acids. ■ Current fat replacers/substitutes approved by the FDA are safe for use in food.
Alcohol	■ If individuals choose to drink, daily alcohol intake should be limited to 1 drink for adult women and 2 drinks for adult men. A 12-oz beer, 5-oz wine, or 1½-oz distilled spirits each equal one drink (each contains ~15 g alcohol). ■ When moderate amounts of alcohol are ingested with food, blood glucose and insulin levels are not affected by alcohol.

(Table 2 continued)

TABLE 2:   Key Nutrition Principles (*continued*)

Nutrient Recommendations for Type 1 and Type 2 Diabetes (1,2) (*continued*)

	■ In individuals using insulin or insulin secretagogues, to reduce the risk of hypoglycemia, alcohol should be consumed with food. Alcoholic beverages are considered an addition to the regular food plan, and no food should be omitted.
Vitamins and minerals	■ There is no clear benefit from supplementation in individuals who do not have underlying deficiencies; exceptions are folate and calcium. ■ Routine supplementation with antioxidants is not advised because of uncertainties related to long-term efficacy and safety.

Nutrition Recommendations for Children and Adolescents with Diabetes (1,2)

MNT objectives for youth with type 1 diabetes	■ Provide adequate energy to ensure normal growth and development. ■ Integrate insulin regimens into usual eating and physical activity habits.
MNT objectives for youth with type 2 diabetes	■ Facilitate changes in eating and physical activity habits that reduce insulin resistance and improve metabolic status.
Food/meal plan	■ In youth with type 1 diabetes, use individualized food/meal plans and flexible insulin regimens and insulin algorithms to accommodate irregular meal times and schedules, varying appetites, and varying physical activity levels. ■ In obese children, encourage increased physical activity, which will improve lipids and insulin sensitivity, and a healthy eating pattern. ■ Nutrient requirements are similar to other school-age children and adolescents.

Nutrition Recommendations for Pregnancy and Lactation (1,2)

MNT objectives for pregnant or lactating women with preexisting diabetes	■ Provide adequate energy and nutrients needed for optimal outcomes (glucose control, good nutrition, weight gain, blood pressure control, and prevention of hypoglycemia). ■ For women planning pregnancy, a food/meal plan and insulin regimen that promotes excellent glucose control decreases potential problems with pregnancy.
Food/meal plan	■ Nutrient requirements during pregnancy and lactation are similar for women with and without diabetes. ■ Adequate energy intake and appropriate distribution of meals and snacks are needed to prevent ketosis; an evening snack may be needed to prevent ketosis overnight.

Nutrition Recommendations for Pregnancy and Lactation (1,2) (*continued*)

	■ Successful lactation requires coordination of care and planning for insulin or food plan adjustments following delivery. ■ Use of nonnutritive sweeteners is safe during pregnancy. ■ Although often prescribed, there is inadequate evidence to support the benefit of prenatal vitamin-mineral supplementation, except for folate and perhaps iron. Supplementation is based on assessment of need.
MNT objectives for women with gestational diabetes	■ Provide food choices for appropriate weight gain, normoglycemia, and absence of ketones. ■ Prevent subsequent development of diabetes. Lifestyle strategies to reduce weight or to prevent weight gain and to increase physical activity after pregnancy (and lactation) are recommended.
Food/meal plan	■ To prevent ketosis, adequate energy intake and appropriate distribution of meals and snacks is important. An evening snack is usually needed. ■ For some women, modest energy and carbohydrate restriction may be appropriate. ■ Use of nonnutritive sweeteners is safe during pregnancy. ■ Regular physical activity can improve glucose intolerance.

Nutrition Recommendations for Older Adults (1,2)

MNT objective for older adults	■ Provide for the nutritional and psychosocial needs of an aging individual.
Food/meal plan	■ Energy requirements for older adults are less than those for younger adults. ■ Physical activity should be encouraged. ■ In the elderly, undernutrition is more likely than overnutrition; therefore, caution should be used when prescribing weight loss diets. ■ Dietary restrictions for elderly residents in long-term care facilities are not warranted. Residents with diabetes should be served regular (unrestricted) menus with consistency in the amount and timing of carbohydrate. ■ There is no evidence to support diets such as "no concentrated sweets" or "no sugar added."

Nutrition Recommendations for Associated Complications (1,2)

Goal	■ Prevent and treat the comorbid conditions of diabetes; modify nutrient intake and lifestyle as appropriate for prevention and treatment of hypertension, dyslipidemia, nephropathy, neuropathy, and catabolic illness.

(Table 2 continued)

TABLE 2: Key Nutrition Principles (*continued*)

Nutrition Recommendations for Associated Complications (1,2) (*continued*)

Hypertension	▪ Reduce daily sodium intake to ≤2400 mg or salt to ≤6 g. ▪ A modest weight loss beneficially affects blood pressure. ▪ Drinking small-to-moderate amounts of alcohol will not adversely affect blood pressure. Excessive amounts of alcohol should be avoided. ▪ A low-fat diet that includes fruits and vegetables (5–9 servings/day) and low-fat dairy products (2–4 servings/day) is rich in potassium, magnesium, and calcium and reduces blood pressure.
Dyslipidemia	▪ Elevated LDL cholesterol: limit saturated fat and trans fat to <10% and perhaps <7% of energy, which if replaced can be substituted by carbohydrates or monounsaturated fats. ▪ Diabetes and metabolic syndrome: improve glycemic control, modest weight loss, restrict saturated fats, increase physical activity, and if weight loss is not a goal, incorporate more monounsaturated fats. ▪ Add plant stanols/sterols and increase soluble fiber to enhance lowering of LDL cholesterol. ▪ Triglycerides >1000 mg/dl: restrict all types of fat (except foods containing omega-3 fats).
Nephropathy	▪ Microalbuminuria: reduce protein to 0.8–1.0 g/kg body weight/day. ▪ Overt nephropathy: lower protein to 0.8 g/kg body weight/day.
Gastric neuropathy	▪ Modify texture and food frequency—use 6 low-fat, low-fiber meals per day. ▪ Injecting insulin postmeal may be helpful for some patients.
Catabolic illness	▪ Hospitalized patients: 25–35 kcal/kg body weight/day ▪ Protein needs are 1.0–1.5 g/kg body weight/day, with the higher end of the range used for more stressed patients, e.g., burn patients.

Lifestyle Recommendations for the Prevention of Diabetes (1,2)

Goal for individuals at risk for diabetes	▪ To decrease risk, encourage physical activity and promote food choices that facilitate moderate weight loss or at least prevent weight gain.
Lifestyle strategies	▪ Sustained modest weight loss of ~5–7% of body weight through reduced fat and energy intake and increased physical activity reduces the risk of developing diabetes. ▪ Structured programs that emphasize lifestyle changes are necessary to accomplish these objectives.

> **Lifestyle Recommendations for the Prevention of Diabetes (1,2) *(continued)***
>
> ■ Regular physical activity should be encouraged for all individuals, especially family members of individuals with type 2 diabetes, to decrease risk of developing type 2 diabetes.
> ■ Increased intake of whole grains and dietary fiber may reduce risk.
> ■ Reduced intake of total fat, particularly saturated fat, may improve insulin sensitivity and reduce risk, independent of weight loss.

Process for Providing Medical Nutrition Therapy

The American Dietetic Association has written and validated by clinical trials nutrition practice guidelines (NPGs) for type 1 diabetes, type 2 diabetes, and gestational diabetes (11). NPGs outline a system or process for providing MNT for patients with diabetes. NPGs recommend that patients with diabetes be referred to a dietitian within the first month of diagnosis (or 1 week if for gestational diabetes). Education is a planned process that requires time, materials, space, and professional expertise to implement. A series of 2–3 visits is recommended totaling approximately 2.5–3 h. Additional follow-up is recommended if further education is needed, medications or insulin have been added to therapy, or follow-up is needed for weight loss. Ongoing self-management education is recommended at 6-month to 1-year intervals. The time needed for the first visit will be 60–90 min with 30–45 min needed for each follow-up visit.

The knowledge and skills needed to implement nutrition guidelines and self-management cannot be acquired in one session, and nutrition self-management education must be an ongoing component of diabetes care. For patients whose diabetes is newly diagnosed, a staged approach to education and implementation should be employed. Initial sessions focus on basic food/eating and physical activity skills that have been prioritized by the health care provider and the individual with diabetes. Chapter 3 includes a table that prioritizes nutrition recommendations. In-depth information, skills, and additional topics are added after patients have had time to adjust to the diagnosis of diabetes. Topics are numerous and vary according to individual characteristics, needs and desires, and type of diabetes.

MNT can be implemented in groups or individually. Chapter 3 discusses implementation of self-management education in groups, and Chapter 4 pertains to individual implementation. Appropriate patients for group sessions are individuals with type 2 diabetes on nutrition therapy only or nutrition therapy combined with oral glucose-lowering medications, individuals with type 1 diabetes beginning insulin and nutrition therapy, and women with gestational diabetes. Groups should be composed of <10 patients, and all should understand and speak the same language.

Patients with diabetes who will benefit from individual sessions include those who require an interpreter, who need a very simplified approach or have other learning barriers, who work rotating shifts, who have complications that require specific nutrition recommendations, whose therapy is being intensified, or who are using an insulin pump.

The American Diabetes Association's position statement "Standards of Medical Care for Patients with Diabetes Mellitus" recommends that people with diabetes should receive individualized MNT as needed to achieve treatment goals, preferably by a registered dietitian familiar with the components of diabetes MNT (12). Individualized food/meal plans should not begin with a predetermined calorie level and macronutrient distribution. It is the responsibility of the dietitian to determine the nutrition prescription based on the food and nutrition assessment. Outcomes must be identified and the effectiveness of nutrition interventions continually evaluated. Responsibilities of the physician or referral source and the dietitian are listed in Table 3 (13).

Both group and individual self-management nutrition education have five components (14):

- assessment for developing the nutrition intervention and prescription
- implementation of self-management education
- establishment of clinical and behavioral goals
- evaluation of outcomes
- documentation

Ongoing education is also essential. At the beginning and throughout the process, the person with diabetes and the health care team must have established rapport if the nutrition intervention is to be successful.

TABLE 3: Physician or Referral Source and Dietitian Responsibilities Related to MNT for Diabetes (13)

Physician or referral source responsibilities	■ Refer patient to dietitian for MNT ■ Provide referral data: diabetes treatment regimen; laboratory data including A1C, fasting plasma glucose, cholesterol fractionations, microalbumin; blood pressure; goals for patient care; medical history; medications that affect MNT; clearance for physical activity. ■ Communicate medical treatment goals to patient and reinforce basic nutrition messages. ■ Based on the outcomes of the nutrition intervention, adjust medications if needed.
Dietitian responsibilities	■ Obtain referral data and treatment goals before the initial nutrition intervention. ■ Determine whether patient has financial coverage for MNT. ■ Obtain and assess food intake, physical activity levels, self-monitoring blood glucose levels, and psychosocial and economic issues. ■ Evaluate patient's knowledge, skill levels, readiness to change, and goals. ■ Determine and implement an appropriate nutrition prescription, and provide self-management education on food/meal planning using appropriate educational materials. ■ Evaluate the effectiveness of MNT on medical outcomes, and adjust MNT as appropriate. ■ Communicate recommendations to the referral source based on the outcomes of nutrition interventions and progress/outcomes to all team members. Evaluation of initial glucose outcomes (A1C) should be done between 6 weeks and 3 months after the initial intervention. ■ Plan for follow-up and ongoing education.

Reimbursement/Coverage

Evidence-based research strongly suggests that MNT provided by a registered dietitian who is experienced in the management of diabetes is clinically effective (15). The lack of reimbursement/coverage has often been a barrier for individuals with diabetes to obtain MNT on an outpatient basis. However, this has improved, and today many people can obtain coverage.

Forty-seven states have passed laws that require health insurance companies, including managed care plans, to cover diabetes skills and self-management training, which includes MNT. These laws do not cover any government programs such as Medicaid or Medicare, or employers' self-funded health plans. The number of large employer health plans and other types of health plans covering MNT is also increasing. A referral and/or letter from a physician, documenting the need for and importance of MNT, can assist in improving reimbursement for MNT services.

At the federal level, legislation was passed enabling MNT for diabetes and renal disease to be covered by Medicare beneficiaries as of January 1, 2002. Registered dietitians can be directly reimbursed for MNT services once they have been issued a Medicare provider number. There are several conditions of payment: the service must be initiated by physician referral, registered dietitians and other nutrition professionals must be qualified providers, and patients with type 1, type 2, or gestational diabetes are eligible for diabetes MNT. Registered dietitians can be directly reimbursed for the service, and new CPT and ICD-9-CM codes for MNT have been designated.

Medicare beneficiaries with diabetes who are eligible can also be covered for a minimal amount (10 h initially and 2 h annually) of outpatient diabetes self-management education (DSME), including MNT. To be eligible for reimbursement, an education program must be approved by a CMS-certified accreditor of diabetes education programs, such as the American Diabetes Association Education Recognition Program, and the referring physician or qualified nonphysician provider must prescribe services. For Medicare reimbursement, group education is recommended. To qualify for individual education, specific education needs should be documented. Figure 1A (Appendix) is a sample referral form that includes an area where specific education needs can be identified for individual education.

It is important to encourage people with diabetes to learn about their benefits and to be proactive in obtaining coverage for MNT and diabetes education.

2

Motivation: Facilitating Behavior Change

Information alone is not enough to result in behavioral changes. The key to effective medical nutrition therapy, including self-management education, is to develop a relationship with patients while finding ways to help them take responsibility for how and when to change their overall eating and activity patterns (16).

Establishing rapport is a crucial first step. Both group and individual sessions are more effective if the sessions begin by determining what the patient wants to know and accomplish and what you can do to be of assistance. Asking patients if they are accomplishing medical goals and comparing target values with the patients' data can also help an individual determine whether making lifestyle changes is important for them. Although medical goals are defined, how they are achieved varies from person to person and must be individualized.

Additionally, asking patients if there are behaviors they can change to assist in meeting their goals can also help to determine the direction of the education session. Asking what is the most difficult aspect of lifestyle to change can generate energy for the session. This is particularly important for individuals who have lived with diabetes for long periods of time and need renewed enthusiasm to continue living well with diabetes.

The Transtheoretical Model of Intentional Behavior Change

People differ in their readiness to make behavior changes. The transtheoretical model, proposed by Ruggiero and Prochaska (17), is a general model of intentional behavior change (Table 4). It includes a sequence of stages along a continuum of behavior change and can be used to help professionals understand their client's readiness to change behaviors.

Different intervention strategies are needed for individuals at different stages of the change process. Many patients are not ready to make dramatic lifestyle changes during an initial encounter. Of people in need of lifestyle change, 80% are reported to be in the precontemplation or contemplation stages (18). Professionals often assume that patients are ready for action when in actuality they are still stuck in precontemplation. Most nutrition education and counseling approaches are targeted to individuals in the preparation and action stages. Motivational interventions may work best with individuals who are in the earlier contemplative stages, whereas specific skill-training interventions may be most appropriate for individuals who have decided to change. Relapse and recycling through the stages occur quite frequently as individuals attempt to modify behaviors (17).

Precontemplation and contemplation. Communication during initial encounters should emphasize information about lifestyle risks and simple, positive lifestyle changes the patient can make to decrease these risks. A discussion about the benefits and barriers to improved glucose control is likely to be of more benefit to individuals in the precontemplation stage than, for example, providing guidelines on how to reduce fat in the

TABLE 4: Transtheoretical Model of Intentional Behavior Change

Stage of Change Model	Attitude Toward Lifestyle Change	Description
Precontemplation	"Never"	■ Individuals have no intention of changing behavior in the foreseeable future. ■ They are usually unaware that they have a problem and are resistant to efforts to modify the behavior.
Contemplation	"Someday"	■ Individuals are aware they have a problem and are seriously thinking about change. ■ However, they have not yet made a commitment to take action in the near future.
Preparation	"Soon"	■ Individuals are at the stage of decision making. ■ A commitment to take action within the next 30 days has been made. ■ Small behavioral changes are already being made.
Action	"Now"	■ Individuals are making notable overt efforts to change. ■ The target behavior has been modified to an acceptable criterion. ■ However, new behaviors may not be consistently carried out.
Maintenance	"Forever"	■ Individuals are working to stabilize their behavior change and to avoid relapse. ■ In general, maintenance is sustaining action for at least 6 months.

Adapted from Ref. 17.

diet. Patients who hold two important beliefs are more likely to begin self-management behaviors than are those who do not have these beliefs (19):

■ They believe diabetes to be serious.
■ They believe that their own actions can make a difference.

The techniques of motivational interviewing given in Table 5 have proved to be helpful for professionals (16).

Preparation and action. A person's self-efficacy and self-confidence in making and maintaining a change is a significant predictor of later adherence (20). Focusing on lifestyle strategies that are feasible and realistic and assuring the patient that he or she can achieve these goals can increase the patient's confidence in his or her ability to make important lifestyle changes.

Behavior modification is a method for systematically modifying eating, exercise, or other behaviors. Techniques that patients who have made lifestyle changes find to be most helpful have been reported. Although this research has not focused solely on individuals with diabetes, individuals making lifestyle changes face similar challenges, and it is likely that strategies that help individuals who struggle with lifestyle changes to control weight will also be helpful to individuals with diabetes. Helpful techniques include self-monitoring, stimulus control, contingency management, cognitive restructuring, and stress management (Table 6)(21).

TABLE 5: Techniques of Motivational Interviewing

Support self-efficacy	■ Provide choices and reassure of expected outcomes
Express empathy	■ Express acceptance and understanding ■ Use reflective listening and expect ambivalence
Explore discrepancies	■ Let individuals explore their reasons for changing or not changing behaviors
Avoid arguments	■ Avoid judging and labeling ■ Change strategies if individuals show resistance
Promote empowerment	■ Individuals are a source of solutions, and because diabetes is a self-managed disease, the individual is in charge and responsible for his or her own care

TABLE 6: Techniques for Modifying Behavior

Self-monitoring	■ Recording of target behaviors and factors associated with behaviors; always reported by participants as most helpful ■ Self-recording of food, exercise, and blood glucose monitoring records
Stimulus control	■ Restricting environmental factors associated with inappropriate behaviors ■ Eating at specific times; setting aside time and place for exercise ■ Avoiding purchasing foods that are difficult to control eating
Contingency management	■ Rewarding appropriate behaviors ■ Contracts used to formalize agreements; contracts should be short term and focus on increasing healthy behaviors
Cognitive restructuring	■ Used to help move thinking patterns away from self-rejection and toward self-acceptance ■ Changing thinking patterns from unrealistic goals to realistic and achievable goals
Stress management	■ Stress is a primary predictor of relapse; therefore, methods to reduce stress and tension are critical. ■ Tension reduction skills include diaphragmatic breathing, progressive muscle relaxation, and/or meditation. ■ Regular exercise helps reduce stress.

Maintenance

Successful self-management involves an ongoing process of problem solving, adjustment, and readjustment. Individuals must be taught how to anticipate and deal with the wide variety of decisions they will face on a daily basis. Furthermore, it is essential that support from family and friends be provided in the right balance; the right amount is important in promoting adherence, but more than the desired amount negatively effects these behaviors (22). Techniques to assist individuals maintain behavior change also have been identified (Table 7)(23).

Medical nutrition therapy that is designed around a patient-centered framework is often more time-consuming and challenging, but its chances for success are greater. Simply delivering information is not enough to ensure action. Patients also need

TABLE 7: Techniques for Maintaining Behavior Changes

Structured programs with frequent patient contact	■ Results from diabetes prevention trials show clearly that just giving information to patients does not result in behavior change. ■ To assist individuals in achieving goals requires structured programs with consistent follow-up contacts. ■ Seeing the diabetes health care team on a regular basis can provide continued education and support.
Social support	■ Social support can be from family or involvement in social activities and is an important component of successful behavior change. ■ Peer support is particularly useful.
Exercise	■ Individuals who exercise regularly are also more likely to maintain other healthy behaviors.
Relapse-prevention training	■ Relapse to inappropriate behaviors tends to occur when the person is alone, under stress, or in social situations. ■ Individuals can practice coping strategies to handle high-risk situations.

Adapted from Ref. 23.

skills to help them make behavioral changes necessary to ensure the goals and effectiveness of MNT. And just as support from family and friends is important, continuing education from professionals is also essential and can provide support for patients' problem-solving skills and decision-making strategies.

3

Implementing Group Medical Nutrition Therapy

Providing MNT in groups is becoming increasingly important. Reimbursement criteria for diabetes self-management education and for MNT for diabetes recommend that, when possible, group sessions are preferable. A group is defined as two or more but less than ten patients. It is helpful if group participants are similar in their stage of diabetes management and if they all speak and understand the same language. Groups are commonly composed of individuals with newly diagnosed type 2 diabetes using MNT only or MNT plus oral glucose-lowering agents, or individuals with type 2 diabetes in need of a review of self-management skills and techniques to improve glycemic control. A major benefit of group education is the support and motivation to change that participants receive from one another. In addition, group members learn from each other and from the discussions of common questions and concerns.

The process for providing group MNT is similar to the process used for implementing individual MNT and involves assessment, intervention including self-management education, goal setting, evaluation, and communication (documentation). However, group education shifts more responsibility to the patient to provide the needed initial assessment information, for the evaluation of outcomes, and for decision-making concerning therapy changes. Because the amount of one-on-one time with the patient is usually limited, assessment tools that the patient can complete before sessions are recommended and a set curriculum followed.

Nutrition practice guidelines recommend that individuals with diabetes be referred to a dietitian within the first month of diagnosis. A series of three visits are recommended, totaling approximately 2.5–3 h (11). Although a nutrition education curriculum is important for groups, the food plan needs to be individualized. Nutrition education often focuses first on carbohydrate because it is the nutrient that affects glucose levels. Consistency in the number of carbohydrate choices at each meal and eating at approximately the same time each day are the first steps for improved glycemia. At the first follow-up session, when food and blood glucose records are available, the food plan can be individualized, i.e., an appropriate number of carbohydrate choices per meal determined.

The suggested topics to be covered at each session are presented in Table 8 (24). Having a planned curriculum ensures continuity if patients find they need to change groups or if instructors change.

First Session

Assessment. Two sets of assessment data are necessary before beginning self-management education and goal setting. The first is data from the referral source (or the patient's medical records), and the second is information from the patient. By collecting these data before the first session, implementation of education can begin efficiently. In the Appendix, there are a sample referral form (Figure 1A) and a sample patient questionnaire (Figure 2A). With the shortened time available for education, it is essential that these data be collected before the session, as the actual assessment time with patients is short.

TABLE 8: Sessions and Suggested Nutrition Educational Topics

First session	■ Brief review of diabetes, management, and therapy goals
	■ Small changes in lifestyle can add up to major improvements in glucose and lipids
	■ Impact of food on glucose
	■ Carbohydrate counting guidelines
	■ How to use Nutrition Facts on food labels
	■ Importance of and guidelines for physical activity
First follow-up session (second visit)	■ Review food and blood glucose records and then individualize food plan
	■ Fat modifications
	■ Treatment of hypoglycemia, if appropriate
	■ Managing sick days
Second follow-up session (third visit)	■ Review lifestyle behaviors
	■ Tips for eating out
	■ Guidelines for use of alcohol
	■ Need for continued education and follow-up

Adapted with permission from Ref. 24.

The following parameters either from the referral source or patient are assessed: laboratory data, food/nutrition history, anthropometric measures, learning style, cultural heritage, and socioeconomic status. Minimum referral data needed from a physician or referral source are listed in Table 9.

The individual's height and weight (and blood pressure) can be done during registration. Body mass index (weight/height^2) can be determined from a chart (see Table 1A in the Appendix).

It is essential to learn about the patient's lifestyle and eating habits. Sending patients a short lifestyle history form to be filled in and brought to the scheduled appointment or scheduling the patient to arrive 15 min early so history forms can be completed saves time and is likely to be as accurate as directly asking patients these questions. (See Figure 2A in the Appendix, which is a sample patient questionnaire for nutrition education.) The data that can be obtained from a lifestyle history form are given in Table 10.

Food/nutrition histories can be done in several ways. Initially asking the individual to record what, how much, and when he or she typically eats during a 24-hour period may be

TABLE 9: Minimum Referral Data Needed for Assessment

Diabetes treatment regimen	■ Nutrition therapy alone ■ Nutrition therapy and oral-glucose lowering agents (type[s]) ■ Nutrition therapy and insulin (fixed or flexible regimen) ■ Nutrition therapy and combination medications (type[s])
Laboratory data	■ A1C, date of test ■ Fasting or nonfasting plasma glucose ■ Lipid fractionation (cholesterol, LDL and HDL cholesterol, triglycerides) ■ Urinary microalbumin (albumin-to-creatinine ratio) ■ Blood pressure
Goals for patient care	■ Target blood glucose levels (pre- and postmeal) ■ Target A1C ■ Method and frequency of self-monitoring of blood glucose (SMBG) ■ Plans for instruction and evaluation of SMBG
Medical history	■ Other pertinent diagnoses: cardiovascular disease, hypertension, renal disease, autonomic neuropathy, especially gastrointestinal ■ Medications for dyslipidemia and blood pressure; other medications
Guidelines for exercise	■ Medical clearance for exercise ■ Exercise limitations, if any

Adapted from Ref 13.

the most useful. This can be a portion of the lifestyle history form such as illustrated in Figure 2A. An alternative approach is to record exactly what was eaten during a specified time period. This provides objective information but may not be a typical day's intake. Figure 3A is an example of a separate 1-day food history form.

Intervention (self-management education). The session might begin with a very brief review of the different types of diabetes, emphasizing that, regardless of the type of diabetes, the goal is to control blood glucose levels. At this point, a review of normal blood glucose levels, patient blood glucose goals, optimal lipids, and blood pressure can occur. (See Table 2A in the

Appendix for the American Diabetes Association goals.) Patients can also compare their lab data to the recommended values. The point is that the overall goal is to employ lifestyle strategies and, when needed, pharmacological therapies that lead to improved and maintained metabolic control (i.e., glucose, lipids, blood pressure).

Explain that MNT (food and activity planning) is important for all treatment options. Treatment options include MNT only, MNT combined with oral glucose-lowering agents, MNT combined with insulin, or MNT combined with several oral agents or oral agents and insulin. MNT is usually used as

TABLE 10: Data to Be Obtained from a Food/Nutrition History Form

Patient demographics	■ Date of birth, ethnicity ■ Occupation, marital status ■ Weight history
Past experiences with nutrition therapy	■ Questions and concerns the patient wishes to have addressed ■ Food/meal planning methods patient is familiar with ■ Percentage of time a food/meal plan is followed ■ Weight history, current weight, recent weight changes, height, body mass index
Schedules/ typical meals/ food concerns	■ Usual meal and eating times ■ Typical day meals and snacks ■ Questions and concerns about food or meal planning ■ Frequency of eating in restaurants ■ Alcoholic beverage usage
Physical activity	■ Usual physical activities ■ Type, frequency, time of day, duration ■ Physical activity limitations
Education/social issues	■ Goals for diabetes management and blood glucose ■ Blood glucose monitoring: frequency, times of day, method ■ Hypoglycemic problems ■ Education barriers ■ Identify a support person
Medication/ supplements	■ Medications currently taken ■ Vitamin/mineral/supplements taken ■ Herbal products used

monotherapy if fasting glucose is <200 mg/dl or if a random (casual) glucose is <250 mg/dl. Treatment options (such as adding oral medications or insulin) change over the course of diabetes management. It should be emphasized that this is not a failure on the part of the patient but a failure of the patient's pancreas to produce adequate insulin as time progresses. Any therapy that is not assisting the patient in reaching treatment goals requires change so that target goals can be reached.

Begin by asking for questions and concerns that patients have in regard to food and meal planning so they can also be addressed. At this point, it is helpful to prioritize diabetes lifestyle strategies (Table 11). Patients in groups will usually have type 2 diabetes, because they are the majority of people with diabetes. If individuals in the group have type 1 diabetes, or require insulin, differences will need to be addressed individually, i.e., before or after group sessions.

At the first session, it is helpful if individuals are given a starting number of carbohydrate choices for meals/snacks. After individuals have had some experience with carbohydrate counting, it is more realistic to individualize. The decision to include snacks is made by the individual, the daily schedule, and the therapy regimen. Individuals may choose to have snacks if they are very hungry between meals, snacks are a part of their lifestyle, usual mealtimes are more than 4–6 hours apart, or individuals are very active. Snacks are generally not needed unless individuals use an insulin that has its peak effect between meals (i.e., regular or NPH insulin). Explaining how to use the information from Nutrition Facts on food labels is also important.

Table 12 can be used to decide on a starting number of carbohydrate choices. These calorie levels are based on 4–6 oz of cooked meats or meat substitute per day and 5–6 fat servings (1 fat serving = 5 g fat) per day. Meat and fat servings will be discussed in the second session.

Table 13 lists examples of food groups that contain carbohydrate and 15-g serving sizes.

Although carbohydrate counting works well for a basic food planning system for nearly all patients with diabetes, some

TABLE 11: Lifestyle Strategies for Type 2 Diabetes and Teaching Points

1. Lifestyle changes will improve blood glucose control. Lipids and blood pressure are also important but are addressed in follow-up sessions.	■ Following a food plan, consistent carbohydrate intake, and being physically active are the first priorities. ■ Energy restriction (eating less food) independent of weight loss improves glycemia. ■ A small amount of weight loss may improve glycemia and lipids in some individuals.

2. Carbohydrate counting controls total carbohydrate, energy intake, and postprandial glucose levels.	■ There are three food groups:
	  ● Carbohydrates
	  ● Meats and meat substitutes
	  ● Fat
	■ Foods containing carbohydrate are important for good nutrition. For glucose control, the amount of carbohydrate eaten, not the type, is most important.
	■ Grouping carbohydrates into one category (instead of separately as starches, fruits, milk, and sweets) simplifies food and meal planning.
	■ 15 g carbohydrate is the basis for 1 carbohydrate serving. The carbohydrate content of foods can be determined from Nutrition Facts on food labels or by knowing the average size of a portion of food containing 15 g carbohydrate. See Table 13 for some examples. An awareness of average portion sizes enables individuals with diabetes to look at a plate of food and estimate how many carbohydrate servings it contains.
	■ Individuals need to know how many carbohydrate servings (or grams) to select for meals and snacks (if desired). See Table 12 for suggested carbohydrate servings per meal.

3. Physical activity improves insulin resistance and lowers blood glucose.	■ Physical activity improves glycemia, decreases insulin resistance, improves risk factors for cardiovascular disease, lowers blood pressure, and assists with weight maintenance. ■ For improved glycemia, physical activity must be repeated on a regular basis. ■ Goal: minimum cumulative total of 1000 kcal/week (1 mile walking = ~100 kcal).

(Table 11 continued)

TABLE 11: Lifestyle Strategies for Type 2 Diabetes and Teaching Points (*continued*)

	■ Short periods of activity throughout the day are beneficial; accumulate 30 min or more every day. ■ For reduced cardiovascular mortality, it is more important to be fit than thin (25).
4. Food and blood glucose monitoring records are used to determine whether lifestyle changes will improve glycemia or if changes in therapy are needed.	■ Emphasize consistency in carbohydrate intake. ■ Evaluate the largest meal by testing both pre- and postprandial glucose values. Goal for postprandial glucose: <160–180 mg/dl 2 h after the start of the meal. ■ Type 2 diabetes is a progressive disease, and the need for changes in medical therapy is not patient failure but a failure of the pancreas to produce adequate amounts of insulin. ■ A1C outcomes will be known by 3 months. If glucose goals are not achieved, adding or changing medications will likely be needed.

Source: International Diabetes Center.

patients may prefer or do better with other systems. Other food planning systems include sample menus, calorie counting, or exchanges. These systems will need to be reviewed with patients individually.

In addition, a modest weight loss (5–10 lb) for individuals with insulin resistance may improve glucose and lipid levels, but weight loss should be viewed as a means to an end rather than an end in itself. For example, a patient who is overweight may choose to work on carbohydrate counting rather than focusing on weight. An overall healthy eating pattern will improve overall health and may also improve glucose control and often results in gradual weight loss.

TABLE 12: Carbohydrate Servings per Meal (grams of carbohydrate)*

	To Lose Weight	To Control Weight	For Active Individuals
Women	3–4 (45–60 g)	4–5 (60–75 g)	5–6 (75–90 g)
Men	4–5 (60–75 g)	5–6 (75–90 g)	6–7 (75–105 g)

*If snacks are desired, subtract carbohydrate servings from a meal.

TABLE 13: Carbohydrate Foods

Carbohydrate Groups	Serving Sizes with 15 g Carbohydrate
Grains, pasta, bread, cereal, rice, beans, and starchy vegetables	■ 1 slice bread ■ 1/2 to 3/4 cup dry cereal or 1/2 cup cooked cereal ■ 1/3 cup cooked pasta or rice ■ 3 cups popcorn ■ 1/2 cup beans or starchy vegetable (peas, corn, mashed potatoes) ■ 1 small potato
Fruit	■ 1 small piece of fruit ■ 1/2 cup canned fruit ■ 1/2 cup juice ■ 1/4 cup dried fruit
Milk, yogurt, and other dairy products	■ 1 cup fat-free milk ■ 1 cup nonfat fruited yogurt with no-calorie sweetener
Sweets (cookies, ice cream)	■ 2 small (2-inch) cookies ■ 1/2 cup ice cream or frozen yogurt ■ 1/4 cup sherbet

Adapted from Ref. 26.

Goal setting. Short-term (days/weeks) behavior goals are usually related to lifestyle changes (i.e., food, physical activity, and self-monitoring of blood glucose) and are determined with the patient at the close of the session. Common self-management behavioral goals are consistent carbohydrate choices for meals and snacks, regular physical activity, correct medication dose (if needed), and monitoring blood glucose as needed. Achievement of goals is considered an outcome of MNT intervention and, therefore, goals must be measurable. Goals must also be specific, written in behavioral language, and realistic for the patient. The following tips can assist patients in setting their goals.

■ Encourage patients to only select two to three goals at a time.
■ Encourage patients to select a goal that will have significant impact on them.

- Encourage patients to select a goal that is realistic for them.
- Encourage patients to set positive goals.

These are examples of specific, realistic behavioral goals.

- I will eat only 1 carbohydrate serving at my bedtime snack every night for 2 weeks.
- I will walk 20 min 5 days a week after dinner for the next month.
- I will check my blood glucose before and 2 h after dinner, then record it in my record book, for 1 week.

Planning for follow-up sessions, evaluation, and communication (documentation). End the session on a positive note. Summarize key points and goals, and express appreciation for the patient's participation. For group sessions to be individualized and to lead to successful outcomes, follow-up sessions are essential. Discuss how and when the next session will occur, and express confidence in their ability to follow through. Request that patients keep 3-day or weekly records for food as well as for physical activity and blood glucose monitoring data. Figure 4A in the Appendix is a sample 3-day food, physical activity, and blood glucose record form. This provides invaluable information for the next session. You may also want to let them know how to contact you if they have questions before the next session.

Documentation of the entire process is essential for communication and reimbursement. Table 14 lists the areas of nutrition intervention that need to be communicated to other team members.

First Follow-Up Session

It is helpful if the first follow-up group session can occur within 2–3 weeks after the initial session. It is recommended that group member composition be kept consistent, although this is not always possible. If a set curriculum is being followed, it is possible for patients to change groups and/or instructors and be assured they are not missing anything.

TABLE 14: First Session Communication and Documentation Areas

- Initial carbohydrate servings for meal and snacks (if patient desires snacks); patient acceptance and understanding of food plan
- Patient's behavioral goals
- Teaching topics to be covered at the next session; additional needed information and skills
- Additional recommendations, comments, or concerns
- Plans for follow-up sessions; make note that you have requested food and blood glucose records to be brought to the next session

Evaluation/assessment. The following areas are evaluated at every visit.

- Food and blood glucose monitoring records
  - Food records are evaluated for consistency in meal times and number of carbohydrate choices per meal/snack.
  - Blood glucose records are evaluated to determine the percentage of readings in the target range. The goal is to have approximately 50% of the readings in range.
- Specific behavior changes per intervention plan
- Schedule changes
- Physical activity patterns
- Weight (height done at initial session)

Food records can be compared with the number of carbohydrate choices initially selected to determine whether the initial food plan is actually feasible for the patient. If the patient has not been able to implement the initial food plan, a more realistic food plan must be developed. Blood glucose monitoring records can be used to determine whether blood glucose values outside the target ranges can be corrected by adjustments in the food plan or whether changes in medication(s) are needed. This assessment can be done in a group discussion encouraging patients to decide what changes are appropriate for them to make, or it can be done quickly individually, perhaps before the session or while weighing the patient.

Figures 5A and 6A in the Appendix, respectively, are samples of an initial food record and an improved food record with carbohydrate servings. Note that by changing portion sizes and making small changes in food servings, not only are the number of carbohydrate choices reduced from 25 to 18 but total kcal, fat, saturated fat, and sodium are reduced as well. Comparing Figures 5A and 6A, you will find the following:

Initial Food Record	Improved Food Record
3300 kcal	2000 kcal
~25 CHO choices	~18 CHO choices
151 g fat (41%)	64 g fat (30%)
64 g saturated fat (17%)	20 g saturated fat (9%)
6450 mg sodium	3900 mg sodium

Intervention (self-management education). After a review of carbohydrate counting, this session can address the role of fat modifications and risk of cardiovascular disease. Review the different types of fatty acids in foods, and provide guidelines on how to lower saturated fat and dietary cholesterol intake. Other suggested topics include sick day management and treatment of hypoglycemia.

By asking the group what questions they have, other topics can be addressed to meet the desires of the group. The education session can end with a review of previous goals and changes or additions the patient wishes to make for the next weeks.

Follow-up and communication. The outcomes from the first follow-up session need to be communicated with other team members. This may be done verbally as well as by updating the initial documentation record.

Second Follow-Up Session

A second follow-up session is recommended within 4–6 weeks, which is approximately 6–12 weeks after the initial session. A second follow-up session is particularly important for patients whose goals have not been met if it is anticipated that changes in medical therapy will be needed, if the patient has had difficulty making lifestyle changes, or if further education is needed. Plans must be made for the patient to have an A1C test before the second follow-up session.

Evaluation/assessment. Food records are reviewed to determine whether the group or individuals understand carbohydrate counting and fat modifications. Goals are reviewed. At this session, it also can be determined whether lifestyle changes are assisting the patient in reaching his or her target glucose ranges or whether changes in therapy will be needed. Changes in therapy should be recommended if

- blood glucose levels or A1C have not shown a downward trend
- patient has lost weight with no improvement in glucose
- patient is doing well with food plan and physical activity, and further nutrition interventions are unlikely to improve medical outcomes

Table 3A in the Appendix contains a list of oral glucose-lowering medications, with their class and generic names, principal site of action, recommended doses, and mean decrease in A1C.

Intervention (continuing self-management education). Information topics to be discussed at this session include strategies for successful eating out, alcohol and its effect on glucose and insulin levels, and, if not covered previously, sick day management and treatment of hypoglycemia. Review treatment options and how and when therapy may need to be advanced. Reinforce lifestyle behavioral goals and the fact that because diabetes is a chronic disease, individuals with diabetes need continued education and support.

Follow-up and documentation. It is suggested that follow-up nutrition care be provided every 6–12 months. This might consist of support groups or individual consults. Finally, communication of outcomes should be documented either in a letter to the referral source or in the patient's medical record.

4

Implementing Individual Medical Nutrition Therapy

Although many individuals with diabetes benefit from group education, there are others who require individual sessions. Those who would benefit from an individualized approach include children, adolescents or adults newly diagnosed with type 1 diabetes, those undergoing diabetes therapy changes, those who require an interpreter or who have a learning handicap, or anyone who needs care before a group appropriate for them is available. However, like group education, the knowledge and skills needed to implement nutrition guidelines cannot be acquired in one session, and MNT must be an ongoing component of diabetes management.

Individual MNT involves a common process—assessment, intervention, evaluation, and communication—working toward the stated medical goals with a personalized intervention, although the medical goals may change slightly because of age, safety, or other reasons. The process begins by establishing rapport with the patient. The intervention is then tailored to the needs of the patient and whether the intervention is for initial, continuing, or intensive care (11). These three factors will also determine the content of the education session and the goals set.

First Session

Assessment. To develop an individualized nutrition care plan and prescription, assess the same parameters as for group self-management education: anthropometric measures, laboratory data, food/nutrition history, learning style, cultural heritage, and socioeconomic status. Minimum referral data include age, diagnosis of diabetes and other pertinent medical history, diabetes-related and other pertinent medications, laboratory data (A1C, cholesterol fractionation, albumin-to-creatinine ratio), blood pressure, and clearance for exercise. See the assessment section in Chapter 3. Table 15 lists the assessments of importance.

Appendix Figure 2A is a sample patient questionnaire for nutrition education that can be used to gather this information. A complete food/history should be taken at the onset of nutrition therapy to familiarize the health care team with the individual's lifestyle and eating habits. A nutrition history form with key questions can be useful for recording the data. Figure 7A in the Appendix is a sample nutrition assessment form.

Food/nutrition histories can be taken in several ways, with the objective being to determine a schedule and pattern of eating that is the least disruptive to the lifestyle of the individuals with diabetes and to determine the insulin regimen that would fit the eating pattern. Just as for group education, asking the individual to either record or to report what, how much, and when he or she typically eats during a 24-hour period may be the most useful. In the Appendix, Figure 3A is a sample 1-day food history form, and Figure 8A is a patient-completed 1-day food intake form.

From the assessment data, a preliminary meal plan can be designed. Figure 1 can be used to record the usual foods eaten and to modify the usual food intake as necessary. The macronutrient and caloric values for the exchange lists are listed on the

TABLE 15: Assessment Issues

Anthropometric measures	■ Weight, height (for adults at initial visit and for children at every visit), BMI
Social history	■ Occupation ■ Hours worked/away from home ■ Living situation ■ Financial issues
Diabetes history	■ Previous diabetes education ■ Use of blood glucose monitoring ■ Diabetes problems/concerns (hypoglycemia, hyperglycemia, fear of insulin)
Food/nutrition history	■ 24-h recall or typical day's intake ■ Meal and snack eating times ■ Schedule changes ■ Travel frequency ■ Exercise routine/sports (type, amount, and time of exercise) ■ Usual sleep habits ■ Appetite/GI issues ■ Food allergies/food intolerance ■ Alcohol use ■ Weight history, weight goals
Medications/ supplements	■ Medications taken ■ Vitamin/mineral/supplement use ■ Herbal supplements

form and are a useful tool for evaluating nutrition assessments. By totaling the number of servings from each list and multiplying the grams of carbohydrate and protein by 4 and the grams of fat by 9, total calories and percentage of calories from each macronutrient can be determined. Figure 9A in the Appendix is a modified meal plan developed from the food history gathered with the form in Figure 8A.

The next step is to evaluate the preliminary meal plan. First and foremost, does the individual with diabetes feel it is feasible to implement? Second, is it appropriate for diabetes management? Third, are the calories appropriate? Fourth, does it encourage healthful eating?

Is the food plan feasible for the individual with diabetes to implement? The food plan is reviewed with the individual in terms of general food intake. Timing of meals and snacks and

FIGURE 1: Food History Form

Time	Bkfst	Snack	Lunch	Snack	Dinner	Snack	Total Servings/ Day	CHO (g)	Protein (g)	Fat (g)	Kcal
Starch								15	3	1	80
Fruit								15			60
Milk								12	8	1	90
Veg								5	2		25
Meat/Sub									7	5(3)	75(55)
Fat										5	45
CHO choices							Total grams				Total =
							Kcal/ gram	×4	×4	×9	
							Percent kcal				

approximate portion sizes and types of foods are covered. A meal-planning approach can be selected to assist the individual in making his or her own food choices. However, at this point, it needs to be determined if this food plan is reasonable for the individual.

Is the food plan appropriate for diabetes management? This involves assessing both distribution of the meals (and snacks, if desired) as well as the macronutrient percentages. Appropriateness is based on the types of medications prescribed as well as the treatment goals.

- For patients on medical nutrition therapy only: The information in Table 16 can be used as a starting point for the number of carbohydrate choices per meal. The individual can do blood glucose checks before and 2 h after the meal, with the plasma glucose goal being premeal values of <130 mg/dl and a 2-h value of <160–180 mg/dl.
- For patients on oral glucose-lowering agents: There are food concerns related to oral agent therapy (Table 17). If the patient is on an insulin secretagogue (i.e., sulfonylureas), meals should not be missed. Individuals with type 2 diabetes do not need snacks unless this is their choice. If they choose to have snacks, they cannot be in addition to the usual meals. A portion of the meal should be saved to be eaten as a snack between meals. See Table 3A in the Appendix for more information on oral glucose-lowering agents.
- For patients on insulin: Table 18 lists points to consider when choosing an insulin regimen. Fixed insulin regimens usually consist of mixtures of short-acting and intermediate-acting insulins (such as regular/NPH) or rapid-acting and intermediate-acting insulins (such as lispro or aspart/NPH) or premixed insulins taken twice a day. Flexible insulin regimens consist of a basal (background) insulin (such as glargine injected once a day or NPH or ultralente injected twice a day) and a

TABLE 16: Carbohydrate Servings for Meals/Snacks (grams of carbohydrate)

Approximate Calories	Meal Servings	Snack Servings per Day (if desired)
1200–1500 (for weight loss)	3 (45 g)	1 (15 g)
1600–2000 (for weight control)	4 (60 g)	2–3 (30–45 g)
2100–2400 (for active individuals)	5 (75 g)	4–6 (60–90 g)

bolus (meal) insulin (such as a rapid-acting insulin) injected before meals. This requires 3–4 injections per day. Types of insulin, onset of action, usual effective duration, and when to monitor the effect of the insulin are listed in Table 4A in the Appendix. For insulin-requiring individuals, the timing of eating is extremely important. Food consumption must be synchronized with the time actions of insulin. Flexible insulin regimens give all patients with either type 1 or type 2 diabetes more options. If the eating pattern is determined first, an insulin regimen can be selected that

TABLE 17: Food Concerns Related to Oral Glucose-Lowering Agents

Biguanides (Glucophage), thiazolidinediones (Actos, Avandia)	■ Recommend the same number of carbohydrate choices per meal as for nutrition therapy alone ■ Agents do not cause hypoglycemia
Sulfonylureas (Amaryl, Micronase)	■ Recommend the same number of carbohydrate choices per meal as for nutrition therapy alone ■ May cause hypoglycemia, and therefore snacks may be needed
Repaglinide (Prandin), nateglinide (Starlix)	■ May be able to eat larger amounts of carbohydrate per meal; this can be determined by checking glucose levels pre- and postmeal
Alpha glucosidase inhibitors (Precose, Glyset)	■ Amount of carbohydrate tolerated will be based on the GI side effects

TABLE 18: Food Concerns Related to Insulin Regimens

Insulin Regimen	Description	Food Issues Related to Insulin Regimen
Fixed insulin regimens	■ Usually 2 injections per day ■ Mixed doses of rapid-acting (lispro or aspart) or short-acting (regular) and longer-acting (NPH or ultralente) insulins ■ Premixed insulins such as 70/30 or 75/25 given at breakfast and supper	■ Consistent meal times are important. ■ If meal times are inconsistent or meals are skipped, this type of insulin regimen does not work well. ■ If short-acting insulin (regular) is combined with intermediate-acting insulin, snacks are helpful. ■ If individuals do not like to snack, a rapid-acting insulin combined with an intermediate- or long-acting insulin is required. ■ Weight loss is often more difficult because individuals need to eat based on the time actions of the insulin injected. ■ When exercising, individuals will often need to add carbohydrate to prevent hypoglycemia. ■ It is helpful to exercise at consistent times.
Flexible insulin regimens	■ Usually 3–4 injections per day ■ Meal time (bolus) insulin dose of rapid- (lispro or aspart) or short-acting (regular) insulin ■ Background (basal) insulin dose of glargine, NPH, or ultralente ■ Insulin pumps	■ Snacks are not needed during the day. An evening snack may be needed. ■ Snacks containing >15 g carbohydrate can be a problem. If larger snacks are eaten, an extra bolus of insulin can be injected presnack. ■ Individuals have the ability to eat less and take less insulin and have more flexibility in the amount of times that food is eaten. As a result, it may be easier to control weight. ■ Insulin can be adjusted to accommodate varying exercise times and amounts of exercise.

will fit with it. The food plan should also be designed to prevent hypo- and hyperglycemia, promote good health and weight, and to manage complications of diabetes (e.g., dyslipidemia, hypertension, renal disease, gastroparesis), as needed.

Table 19 is a summary of how to use eating patterns to determine the insulin regimen.

Does the intake look realistic? Are the kcal appropriate? Next determine whether the number of kcal is appropriate or realistic for the individual. Energy requirements depend on several factors, such as age, gender, height, weight, and activity level. Table 20 outlines a simple method for determining approximate energy requirements based on current weight.

Methods for determining energy requirements are only approximate. On a practical basis, however, they do provide a starting point for evaluating the caloric adequacy of the food plan. Adjustments in calories can be made during follow-up visits. Parameters that should be considered are weight changes, feelings of satiety and hunger, and concerns about palatability.

The determination of a calorie level and a nutrition prescription for a child or adolescent is based on the nutrition assessment. Energy needs can be calculated in various ways (Table 21). However, the best method is to ascertain what the child usually eats to maintain his or her weight, because chil-

Table 19: Using Eating Patterns to Choose Insulin Regimen

If the Patient Prefers	Recommend the Following Insulin Regimen
3 meals, no snacks	■ Flexible insulin regimens using rapid-acting insulin before meals with basal insulin ■ Fixed insulin regimen, but may need evening snack
3 meals, 2 or 3 snacks	■ Fixed insulin regimens using short-acting (regular) with intermediate or long-acting insulin or 70/30
Inconsistent/erratic eating schedule	■ Flexible insulin regimens using rapid-acting insulin (lispro or aspart) before meals with basal insulin

TABLE 20: Estimating Approximate Energy Requirements for Adults

Obese or very inactive individuals and chronic dieters	■ 10–12 kcal/lb (20 kcal/kg)
Individuals >55 years, active women, sedentary men	■ 13 kcal/lb (25 kcal/kg)
Active men, very active women	■ 15 kcal/lb (30 kcal/kg)
Thin or very active men	■ 20 kcal/lb (40 kcal/kg)

dren have a natural ability to know how much to eat for normal growth and development. It is essential that the meal plan for children and adolescents with type 1 diabetes provides sufficient calories. Adolescents and parents of young children need to learn to adjust insulin intake rather than restrict food to control blood glucose levels. For children or adolescents with type 2 diabetes, promote the minimum caloric needs, a lower fat intake, and increase physical activity. Recording height and weight on growth charts assists in determining appropriateness of energy levels.

Does the food plan encourage healthful eating? The best way to ensure nutritional adequacy is to encourage patients to eat a variety of foods from all the food groups. The Food Guide Pyramid (27), with its suggested number of servings from each food group, can be used to compare an individual's food plan with the nutrition recommendations for all Americans.

TABLE 21: Estimating Minimum Energy Requirements for Youth

Age 1 year	■ 1,000 kcal for the first year
Age 2–11 years	■ Add 100 kcal/year to 1000 kcal up 2000 kcal at age 10
Girls ages 12–15 years	■ 2000 kcal plus 50–100 kcal/year after age 10
Girls >15 years	■ Calculate as for an adult (Table 20)
Boys ages 12–15 years	■ 2000 kcal plus 200 kcal/year after age 10
Boys >15 years	■ Sedentary: 16 kcal/lb (30–35 kcal/kg) Moderate physical activity: 18 kcal/lb (40 kcal/kg) Very physically active: 23 kcal/lb (50 kcal/kg)

Intervention. For many patients whose diabetes is newly diagnosed, a staged approach to education is needed, and this is often best done individually. Initial education focuses on the skills needed for survival. Additional topics and in-depth information can be addressed after the individual has had time to adjust to the diagnosis of diabetes. Topics are numerous and vary according to the type of diabetes and the individual characteristics and needs of the patient with diabetes. Table 22 lists basic or survival skills for all individuals with diabetes.

With individual education, an appropriate food-planning approach can be selected and strategies for behavior change that enhance motivation and adherence to necessary lifestyle changes identified. A number of food-planning approaches are available. They range from simple guidelines to more complex counting methods. None of the food-planning approaches has been shown to be more effective than any other, and the tool selected depends on a patient's stage of learning and his or her needs. Table 23 provides brief summaries of various approaches to food planning.

Goal setting. Just as for group self-management education, the individual with diabetes and the professional should mutually identify specific behavioral goals. Patient's interests and concerns can be discerned from the assessment form and specific short-term behavioral goals reviewed at the end of each session. Goals should be realistic and specific. In general, no more than two or three behavioral goals should be identified at one time.

TABLE 22: Basic and Initial Nutrition Therapy: Self-Management Education Survival Skills

- Basic food/meal plan guidelines
- Blood glucose monitoring skills, if not already known
- Signs, symptoms, treatment, and prevention of hypoglycemia if on insulin or insulin secretagogues
- Guidelines for short-term illness management
- Guidelines for exercising safely, if appropriate
- Plans for continuing nutrition care

Adapted from Ref. 13.

TABLE 23: Food-Planning Approaches for Diabetes

Carbohydrate counting	■ *Basic Carbohydrate Counting* (American Diabetes Association and American Dietetic Association) can be used as a basic meal-planning approach for anyone with diabetes. It is based on the concept that after eating, carbohydrate in foods has the major impact on blood glucose levels. One carbohydrate serving is based on the amount of food that contributes 15 g of carbohydrate.
	■ *Advanced Carbohydrate Counting: Using Insulin-to-Carbohydrate Ratios* (American Diabetes Association and American Dietetic Association) is for individuals who have chosen flexible insulin regimens or an insulin pump. The relationship between carbohydrate eaten and insulin injected can be shown as an insulin-to-carbohydrate ratio. This ratio gives the individual a good idea of how much rapid-acting insulin is needed when eating more or less carbohydrate than usual. However, before insulin ratios can be established, blood glucose levels must be under good control and the usual dose of both the basal and rapid-acting insulin determined. The grams of carbohydrate consumed at a meal are divided by the number of units of insulin needed to maintain target glucose goals. This is called an insulin-to-carbohydrate ratio. For example, 75 g carbohydrate may require 8 units rapid-acting insulin, and the insulin-to-carbohydrate ratio would be 1:10. Therefore, for each anticipated addition of 10 g carbohydrate, an additional 1 unit rapid-acting insulin is needed (or for 10 g less of carbohydrate, 1 less unit rapid-acting insulin is needed).
	■ *My Food Plan* (International Diabetes Center) combines both carbohydrate counting and calorie control in a simplified approach. It groups carbohydrate, meat, and fat choices by approximate portion sizes. A form for filling in an individualized meal plan is included.
Simplified approaches	■ *The First Step in Diabetes Meal Planning* (American Diabetes Association and American Dietetic Association) is a pamphlet that promotes healthy eating. It is designed to be given to patients to use until an individualized meal plan can be implemented.
	■ *Healthy Food Choices* (American Diabetes Association and American Dietetic Association) is a pamphlet that promotes healthy eating. It is divided into two sections: guidelines for making healthy food choices, and simplified Exchange Lists.
	■ *Eating Healthy Foods* (American Diabetes Association and American Dietetic Association) is a booklet designed specifically for individuals with minimal reading skills. The amount of text is limited, symbols and color codes are used, and concepts and foods are presented visually.

(Table 23 continued)

TABLE 23: Food-Planning Approaches for Diabetes (*continued*)

	■ *Healthy Eating for People with Diabetes* (International Diabetes Center) is based on the plate method, which visualizes kinds and amounts of food and is used to illustrate portions of common foods in relation to plate size. General guidelines for choosing healthy foods, lowering fat intake, and timing of meals and snacks are included.
Menu approaches	■ *Month of Meals: Classic Cooking, Old-Time Favorites, Meals in Minutes, Vegetarian Pleasures, and Ethnic Delights* (American Diabetes Association) are five books, each containing 28 days of complete menus for breakfast, lunch, dinner, and snacks. They are designed to help patients who need help in planning basic menus for their diabetes.
Exchange Lists approaches	■ *Exchange Lists for Meal Planning* (American Diabetes Association and American Dietetic Association) contains lists that group foods in measures that contribute approximately the same number of calories, carbohydrate, protein, and fat. Foods are divided into 3 basic lists: carbohydrates, meat and meat substitutes, and fat. An individualized food plan that outlines the number of servings from each list for each meal and for snacks is included.

It may also be determined that other referrals are needed. See the goal setting section in Chapter 3, page 31.

Before the patient leaves, the initial session plans and an appointment for a follow-up session should be determined. In making plans for follow-up, begin by asking the patient to keep a 3-day or weekly food record with blood glucose data. Figure 4A in the Appendix is a sample 3-day food, physical activity, and blood glucose record form.

Evaluation and documentation. The effectiveness of the nutrition intervention should be evaluated throughout the entire education process. Table 24 lists items that should be documented after an MNT visit. Figure 10A in the Appendix is a sample documentation form that can be included in the patient's medical record or in a letter to the referral source.

TABLE 24: Documentation Items

Documentation of each MNT visit should include	▪ Patient name and identification information ▪ Date of MNT visit and amount of time spent with patient ▪ Reason for visit ▪ Level of complexity of care (if billing Medicare) ▪ Patient's current diagnosis (and relevant past diagnoses) ▪ Pertinent test results and current medications (name, dose) ▪ Names of others present during MNT ▪ Physician's referral for MNT (if billing Medicare)

Summaries of	▪ Histories: nutrition, medical, social, and family
	▪ Nutrition assessment
	▪ Nutrition problem list
	▪ MNT intervention provided
	  ● Food/meal plan
	  ● Educational topics covered
	▪ Short- and long-term goals
	▪ RD's impressions, patient progress
	  ● Patient acceptance and understanding
	  ● Anticipated compliance
	  ● Successful behavior changes
	▪ Plan of care
	  ● Additional needed skills or information
	  ● Additional recommendations
	  ● Plans for ongoing care

Follow-Up Visits and Continuing Medical Nutrition Therapy

Evaluation. Successful nutrition therapy involves a process of assessment, problem solving, adjustment, and readjustment. Each session begins with an assessment of what direction and information the patient feels will be helpful for him or her. Success at or barriers to meeting behavioral goals identified in the previous session are reviewed. Food records are compared with the food plan to assess whether the initial food plan was feasible for the patient to implement and whether medical goals are being met.

Intervention. In the long term, individuals and team members need to understand that diabetes is a chronic disease and individuals with diabetes need continued or follow-up nutrition care. A patient-centered or empowerment approach can improve adherence to nutrition therapy and occurs in two phases— initial and continuing. As discussed above, initial education provides the information needed at the time of diagnosis, when the patient's treatment program or lifestyle changes, or at the time of initial contact with a patient. Initial skill topics provide information about basic nutrition, diabetes nutrition guidelines, and beginning strategies for altering eating patterns.

Continuing self-management education includes both management skills and lifestyle changes. Continuing education provides essential information for ongoing nutrition self-management. Topics emphasized or chosen are based on the patient's choice, lifestyle, level of nutrition knowledge, and experience in planning, purchasing, and preparing foods and meals. Flexibility in food planning is always addressed. Table 25 lists essential nutrition topics for self-management that can be addressed when appropriate or when needed.

Evaluation/documentation and plans for follow-up. Identified outcomes can be monitored after the second or third visit (approximately 6 weeks after the initial nutrition consult) to determine whether the individual is making progress toward personal goals. If no progress is evident, the individual and educator need to reassess and consider possible revisions to the nutrition care plan. If the patient has done all that she or he can do or is willing to do and blood glucose levels are not in the target range, the referral source should be notified that medications need to be added or adjusted.

TABLE 25: Nutrition Topics for Continuing Self-Management Education

Management skills (information required to make decisions to achieve management goals)
- Food sources of carbohydrate, protein, fat
- How to use Nutrition Facts on food labels
- Food planning (and insulin adjustments) for
  - Short-term illness
  - Delay or changes in meal times
  - Drinking alcoholic beverages
  - Exercise
  - Travel
  - Competitive athletes
  - Holidays
- Treatment and prevention of hypoglycemia
- How to use blood glucose monitoring data for problem-solving and identification of blood glucose patterns
- Behavior change strategies
- Vitamin, mineral, other nutritional supplements
- Working rotating shifts, if needed

Improvement of lifestyle (problem-solving skills)
- Eating away from home
- Eating lunch in school cafeterias
- Fast-food choices
- Grocery shopping guidelines
- Reducing and modifying fat intake
- Reducing sodium/salt use
- New ideas for snacks
- Vegetarian food choices
- Ethnic foods
- Use of convenience foods
- Recipes, menu ideas, cookbooks

Adapted from Ref. 13.

References

1. American Diabetes Association: Evidence-based nutrition principles and recommendations for the treatment and prevention of diabetes and related complications (Position Statement). *Diabetes Care* 25 (Suppl. 1):S50–60, 2002
2. Franz MJ, Bantle JP, Beebe CA, Brunzell JD, Chiasson J-L, Garg A, Holzmeister LA, Hoogwerf B, Mayer-Davis E, Mooradian A, Purnell JQ, Wheeler M: Evidence-based nutrition principles and recommendations for the treatment and prevention of diabetes and related complications (Technical Review). *Diabetes Care* 25:148–98, 2002
3. Kulkarni K, Castle G, Gregory R, Holmes A, Leontos C, Powers M, Snetselaar L, Splett P, Wylie-Rosett J, for the Diabetes Care and Education Dietetic Practice Group: Nutrition practice guidelines for type 1 diabetes mellitus positively affect dietitian practices and patient outcomes. *J Am Diet Assoc* 98:62–70, 1998
4. United Kingdom Prospective Diabetes Study Group: UK Prospective Diabetes Study 7: Response of fasting plasma glucose to diet therapy in newly presenting type II diabetic patients. *Metabolism* 39:905–12, 1990

5. Franz MJ, Monk A, Barry B, McLain K, Weaver T, Cooper N, Upham P, Bergenstal R, Mazze RS: Effectiveness of medical nutrition therapy provided by dietitians in the management of non-insulin-dependent diabetes mellitus: a randomized, controlled clinical trial. *J Am Diet Assoc* 95:1009–17, 1995

6. Delahanty LM, Halford BH: The role of diet behaviors in achieving improved glycemic control in intensively treated patients in the Diabetes Control and Complications Trial. *Diabetes Care* 16:1453–58, 1993

7. Yu-Poth S, Zhao G, Etherton T, Naglak M, Jonnalagadda S, Kris-Etherton PM: Effects of the National Cholesterol Education Program's Step I and Step II dietary intervention programs on cardiovascular disease risk factors: a meta-analysis. *Am J Clin Nutr* 69:632–46, 1999

8. Cutler JA, Follmann D, Allender PS: Randomized trials of sodium restriction: an overview. *Am J Clin Nutr* 65 (Suppl. 1):643S–51S, 1997

9. Stamler R, Stamler J, Gosch FC, Civinelli J, Fishman J, McKeever P, McDonald A, Dyer AR: Primary prevention of hypertension by nutritional-hygienic means: final report of a randomized, controlled trial. *JAMA* 262:1801–807, 1989

10. Sacks FM, Svetkey LP, Vollmer WM, Appel LJ, Bray GA, Harsha D, Obarzanek E, Conlin PR, Miller ER, Simons-Morton DG, Karanja N, Lin P-H for the DASH-Sodium Collaborative Research Group: Effects on blood pressure of reduced dietary sodium and the Dietary Approaches to Stop Hypertension (DASH) diet. *N Engl J Med* 344: 3–10, 2001

11. American Dietetic Association: Nutrition practice guidelines for type 1 and type 2 diabetes and gestational diabetes. CD-ROM. Chicago, American Dietetic Association, 2001

12. American Diabetes Association: Standards of medical care for patients with diabetes mellitus (Position Statement). *Diabetes Care* 25 (Suppl. 1):S33–49, 2002

13. Monk A, Barry B, McClain K, Weaver T, Cooper M, Franz MJ: Practice guidelines for medical nutrition therapy provided by dietitians for persons with non-insulin-dependent diabetes mellitus. *J Am Diet Assoc* 95:999–1006, 1995
14. Tinker LF, Heins JM, Holler HJ: Commentary and translation: 1994 nutrition recommendations for diabetes. *J Am Diet Assoc* 94:507–11, 1994
15. Pastors JG, Warshaw H, Daly A, Franz M, Kulkarni K: The evidence for the effectiveness of medical nutrition therapy in diabetes management. *Diabetes Care* 25:608–13, 2002
16. Shinitzky HE, Kub J: The art of motivating behavior change: the use of motivational interviewing to promote health. *Publ Health Nurs* 18:178–85, 2001
17. Ruggiero L, Prochaska JO (Eds.): Readiness for change: application of the transtheoretical model to diabetes. *Diabetes Spectrum* 61:21, 1993
18. Prochaska JO, Velicer WF: The transtheoretical model of health behavior change. *Am J Health Promotion* 12:38–48, 1997
19. Glasgow RE: Using interactive technology in diabetes self-management. In *Practical Psychology for Diabetes Clinicians*. 2nd ed. Anderson BJ, Rubin RR, Eds. Alexandria, VA, American Diabetes Association, 2002, pp. 51–62
20. Kavanagy DJ, Gooley S, Wilson PH: Prediction of adherence and control in diabetes. *J Behav Med* 16:509–22, 1993
21. Foreyt JP, Goodrick GK: Evidence for success of behavior modification in weight loss and control. *Ann Intern Med* 119:698–701, 1993
22. Boehn S, Schlenk EA, Funnell MM, Powers H, Ponis DL: Predictors of adherence to nutrition recommendations in people with NIDDM. *Diabetes Educ* 23:157–65, 1997
23. Foreyt JP, Goodrick GK: Factors common to successful therapy for the obese patient. *Med Sci Sports Exerc* 23:292–97, 1991

24. Rickheim P, Flader J, Carstensen KM: *Type 2 Diabetes BASICS.* Minneapolis, MN, IDC Publishing, 2000
25. Lee DC, Blair SN, Jackson AS: Cardiorespiratory fitness, body composition, and all-cause and cardiovascular disease mortality in men. *Am J Clin Nutr* 69:373–80, 1999
26. *My Food Plan.* Minneapolis, MN, IDC Publishing, 2000
27. U.S. Department of Agriculture: *The Food Guide Pyramid.* USDA's Human Nutrition Information Service, Hyattsville, MD, 1992

Appendix

FIGURE 1A: Sample Referral Form

Name _____

Address _____

City _____ State _____ Zip _____

Diabetes dx: Type 1 _____ Type 2 _____ Mo/yr diagnosed _____

Reason for referral: New-onset diabetes _____ Uncontrolled diabetes _____

   Insulin start _____ Refresher _____ Hypertension _____ Lipids _____

   IGT_____ Other _____

Specific education needs: Vision _____ Language _____ Hearing _____

   Physical challenge _____ Other (please specify) _____

Target goals for BG and A1C _____

Any restrictions regarding exercise _____

   If none, please initial here for medical clearance for exercise _____

Diabetes medications   None _____

                      Oral glucose-lowering agent (s) _____

                      Insulin regimen _____

                      Other relevant meds _____

Lab data: A1C _____ FPG _____ Microalbumin _____

       Cholesterol _____ HDL _____ LDL _____

       Triglycerides _____ Blood pressure _____

Comments _____

Date _____ Physician signature _____

                     Address _____

                     City, State, Zip_____

                     Telephone number_____

                     Fax number _____

FIGURE 2A: Patient Questionnaire for Nutrition Education

Name _____

What two main food or eating questions do you want answered today?

1 _____

2 _____

What have you been told about food/eating and diabetes? _____

_____

Please tell us what you eat in a typical day:

Time _____ Breakfast or first meal _____

_____

Time _____ Snack _____

Time _____ Lunch or second meal _____

_____

Time _____ Snack _____

Time _____ Dinner or third meal _____

_____

_____

Time _____ Snack _____

How would you describe your appetite?   ☐ Good   ☐ Fair   ☐ Poor

Who prepares meals in your home? _____

How many meals do you eat away from home each week? _____

What food planning method do you use?   ☐ None   ☐ Carbohydrate counting
☐ Exchange Lists ☐ Calorie counting ☐ Healthy eating using the Food Pyramid

How much of the time are you able to follow it?

  ☐ 0–25% ☐ 25–50% ☐ 50–75% ☐ 75–100%

Has your weight changed in the last year?   ☐ No   ☐ Gained   ☐ Lost

What do you think is a realistic weight for you? _____

Do you drink alcoholic beverages?   ☐ Yes   ☐ No

 If yes, what? _____ How many per week? _____

Do you take vitamins or herbal supplements?   ☐ Yes   ☐ No

 If yes, please list _____

Do you exercise now?   ☐ No   ☐ Yes   What do you do? _____

 If you do not exercise now, what activities would you consider? _____

TABLE 1A: Determining Body Mass Index (BMI)

How to use this chart:
1. Find height (in feet and inches) in the left column.
2. Look across the row to find weight (in pounds).
3. Find the number at the top of the column to determine BMI.

BMI	19	20	21	22	23	24	25	26	27*	28	29	30	35	40
							Weight							
4'10"	91	96	100	105	110	115	119	124	129	134	138	143	167	191
4'11"	94	99	104	109	114	119	124	128	133	138	143	148	173	198
5'	97	102	107	112	118	123	128	133	138	143	148	153	179	204
5'1"	100	106	111	116	122	127	132	137	143	148	153	158	185	211
5'2"	104	109	115	120	126	131	136	142	147	153	158	164	191	218
5'3"	107	113	118	124	130	135	141	146	152	158	163	169	197	225
5'4"	110	116	122	128	134	140	145	151	157	163	169	174	204	232
5'5"	114	120	126	132	138	144	150	156	162	168	174	180	210	240
5'6"	118	124	130	136	142	148	155	161	167	173	179	186	216	247
5'7"	121	127	134	140	146	153	159	166	172	178	185	191	223	255
5'8"	125	131	138	144	151	158	164	171	177	184	190	197	230	262
5'9"	128	135	142	149	155	162	169	176	182	189	196	203	236	270
5'10"	132	139	146	153	160	167	174	181	188	195	202	207	243	278
5'11"	136	143	150	157	165	172	179	186	193	200	208	215	250	286
6'	140	147	154	162	169	177	184	191	199	206	213	221	258	294
6'1"	144	151	159	166	174	182	189	197	204	212	219	227	265	302
6'2"	148	155	163	171	179	186	194	202	210	218	225	233	272	311
6'3"	152	160	168	176	184	192	200	208	216	224	232	240	279	319
6'4"	156	164	172	180	189	197	205	213	221	230	238	246	287	328

BMI = weight/height².

FIGURE 3A: Sample 1-Day Food History Form

1-Day Food Record

Name _____ Date _____

Write down everything you had to eat on a typical day. Include all meals and
snacks and the amount eaten.

Time	Food and Beverages	Amount	Method of Preparation	Do Not Write in This Space
Breakfast				
Snack				
Lunch				
Snack				
Dinner				
Evening				

Adapted from Ref. 24.

TABLE 2A: Clinical Goals for Medical Nutrition Therapy in Diabetes (12)

Glycemic Control for People with Diabetes

	Normal	Goal	Additional Action Suggested
Plasma values*			
Average preprandial glucose (mg/dl)	<110	90–130	<90/>150
Average bedtime glucose (mg/dl)	<120	110–150	<110/>180
2 h after the start of the meal (mg/dl)[†]	<140	<160	>180
Whole blood values[‡]			
Average preprandial glucose (mg/dl)	<100	80–120	<80/>140
Average bedtime glucose (mg/dl)	<110	100–140	<100/>160
2 h after the start of the meal (mg/dl)[†]	<130	<150	<170
A1C (%)[§]	<6	<7	>8

*Values calibrated to plasma glucose (check BG meter to see if this is done automatically).
[†] These recommendations come from consensus among diabetes care providers. No American Diabetes Association recommendation exists for postprandial glucose levels.
[‡] Measurement of capillary blood glucose.
[§] A1C is referenced to a nondiabetic range of 4.0–6.0%.

Target Lipid and Blood Pressure Goals for Adults with Diabetes

Total cholesterol (mg/dl)	<200
LDL cholesterol (mg/dl)	<100
HDL cholesterol (mg/dl)	>45 for men >55 for women
Triglycerides (mg/dl)	<150
Blood pressure (mmHg)	<130/<80

FIGURE 4A: Sample Food, Physical Activity, and Blood Glucose Record Form

3-Day Food and Blood Glucose Record Breakfast Example

Name _____ Date _____

* In the upper left-hand corner, record the time of eating
* Underneath the time, record your medication dose(s)
* In the center, write down everything you eat and drink with the amount eaten
* In the upper right-hand corner, record the number of carbohydrate (CHO) servings
* In the bottom left-hand corner, record blood glucose (BG) before eating
* In the bottom right-hand corner, record blood glucose 2 hours after starting eating
* In the last column, write down physical activity, time, type, how long

Breakfast Example

Time: 7:30   CHO choices: 4½
Dose: 6 lispro

1½ cup cornflakes
½ cup skim milk
½ cup orange juice
1 slice toast
1 tsp margarine

BG Before: 152   BG After: 186

Breakfast	Snack	Lunch	Snack	Dinner	Snack	Activity
Time: CHO servings: Dose:	CHO servings:	Time: CHO servings: Dose:	CHO servings:	Time: CHO servings: Dose:	CHO servings:	
BG Before: BG After:		BG Before: BG After:		BG Before: BG After:	BG Before:	
Time: CHO servings: Dose:	CHO servings:	Time: CHO servings: Dose:	CHO servings:	Time: CHO servings: Dose:	CHO servings:	
BG Before: BG After:		BG Before: BG After:		BG Before: BG After:	BG Before:	
Time: CHO servings: Dose:	CHO servings:	Time: CHO servings: Dose:	CHO servings:	Time: CHO servings: Dose:	CHO servings:	
BG Before: BG After:		BG Before: BG After:		BG Before: BG After:	BG Before:	

Adapted from Ref. 24.

FIGURE 5A: First Sample Completed 1-Day Food History Form

1-Day Food Record

1-day food record for Chris: 50 years old, type 2 diabetes for 5 years, 5'8" and 225 lb (BMI 34.5), lost 10 lb after diagnosis, weight stable for last 4 years, inactive. Therapy: medical nutrition therapy. A1C 8.0%.

Name __Chris Jones_____ Date __Jan 10_____

Write down everything you had to eat on a typical day. Include all meals and snacks and the amount eaten.

Time	Food and Beverages	Amount	Method of Preparation	Do Not Write in This Space
Breakfast 7:30	Raisin Bran Toast Orange juice Milk, 2% Peanut butter Margarine Coffee	1 cup 1 slice 10 oz 1 cup		7–8 CHO
Snack 10:00	Coffee	2 cups		
Lunch 12:30	Sandwich Bread Ham and cheese Chips Carrots Apple Diet soft drink	2 slices 1½ oz 1	With mayo	5–6 CHO
Snack	Milk Way	1		1–2 CHO
Dinner 6:00	Pasta, sauce Bread Salad Milk, 2% Meat balls	2 cups 2 slices 1 1 cup	With margarine With dressing	7–8 CHO
Evening 10:30	Ice cream	1 cup		2 CHO

3300 kcal
~25 CHO choices
151 g fat (41%)
64 g saturated fat (17%)
6450 mg sodium

FIGURE 6A: Improved 1-Day Food Record

1-Day Food Record

Name **Chris Jones** _____ Date **Jan 20** _____

Write down everything you had to eat on a typical day. Include all meals and snacks and the amount eaten.

Time	Food and Beverages	Amount	Method of Preparation	Do Not Write in This Space
Breakfast 7:30	Raisin Bran Orange juice Milk, skim Coffee	1 cup 4 oz 1 cup		5 CHO
Snack 10:00	Coffee	2 cups		
Lunch 12:30	Sandwich Bread Ham, no cheese Chips Carrots Apple Diet soft drink	2 slices 3 oz 1 pkg (⅛ oz) 1	With light mayo	4–5 CHO
Snack 3:00	Raisins	2 tbsp		1 CHO
Dinner 6:00	Pasta, sauce Bread Salad Meat balls Margarine	1½ cups 1 slices 4 small 2 tsp	With margarine With light dressing	4–5 CHO
Evening 10:30	Ice cream, light	1 cup		2 CHO

2000 kcal
~18 CHO choices
64 g fat (30%)
20 g saturated fat (9%)
3900 mg sodium

TABLE 3A: Oral Glucose-Lowering Medications

Class and Generic Names	Recommended Dose	Principal Site of Action	Mean Decrease in A1C
Sulfonylureas (second generation) Glipizide (Glucotrol) Glipizide (Glucotrol XL) Glyburide (Glynase Prestabs) Glimepiride (Amaryl)	2.5–20 mg single or divided dose; single dose for XL 12 mg 4 mg	Stimulate insulin secretion from beta cells	1–2%
Meglitinide Repaglinide (Prandin) Nateglinide (Starlix)	0.4–4.0 mg before meals 120 mg before meals	Stimulate insulin secretion from beta cells	1–2%
Biguanide Metformin (Glucophage) Metformin Extended Release (Glucophage XR) Glyburide/metformin (Glucovance; 1.25/250 mg)	500–850 mg tid or 1000 mg bid 500–2000 mg once daily 2.5/500 mg to 5.0/500 mg	Decrease hepatic glucose production; also increases insulin secretion	1.5–2%
Thiazolidinediones Pioglitazone (Actos) Rosiglitazone (Avandia)	15–45 mg daily 4–8 mg daily	Improve peripheral insulin sensitivity	1–2%
Alpha glucosidase inhibitors Acarbose (Precose) Miglitol (Glyset)	25–100 mg tid 25–100 tid	Delay carbohydrate absorption	0.5–1%

FIGURE 7A: Nutrition Assessment Form

Name _____ Age _____ Date _____
Diagnosis of diabetes _____ Present diabetes treatment _____ Dietitian _____
Medical history _____ Other medications _____ Physician _____

Lab Data

A1C _____ BG _____
Cholesterol _____ HDL-C _____
Triglycerides _____ LDL-C _____
BP _____ Microalbumin _____

Target Goals

Target BGs _____ mg/dl to _____ mg/dl
Target A1C _____ %

Other _____

SMBG: Frequency _____ Times of day _____ Method _____
Medical clearance for exercise: Y / N _____ **Exercise limitations** _____

Time	Bkfst	Snack	Lunch	Snack	Dinner	Snack	Total servings/day	CHO (g)	Protein (g)	Fat (g)	Calories
Starch								15	3	1	80
Fruit								15			60
Milk								12	8	1	90
Veg								5	2		25
Meat/Sub									7	5(3)	75(55)
Fat										5	45
Other								Total g			Total =
								Calories %Kcal	×4	×4	×9	

Ht _____ BMI _____ Wt history _____
Wt _____ Reasonable wt _____
Estimated calorie expenditure + Activity factor = Total calorie needs

History

Occupation _____ Hours worked _____
Lives with _____ Meal preparation _____
Hypoglycemia _____ Eating out _____
Schedule changes/weekends/school schedule _____
Exercise: type/frequency _____
Appetite/GI problems/allergies/intolerances _____
Vitamin and mineral supplements _____
Psychosocial/economic _____

Assessment

Goals (nutrition/exercise/SMBG)

Reprinted with permission from the International Diabetes Center, Minneapolis, MN.

FIGURE 8A: Second Sample Completed 1-Day Food History Form

1-Day Food Record

Name Betty Jones   Date Jan 4

Write down everything you had to eat on a typical day. Include all meals and snacks and the amount eaten.

Time Food Is Eaten	Food and Beverages	Amount	Method of Preparation	Do Not Write in This Space
Time you get up 7:00	Orange juice	1 cup		2 fruit
Breakfast 7:30	Corn flakes Milk, 2% Coffee	Large bowl 1 cup 2 cups		2 starch 1 milk 1 fat (5 CHO)
Snack 10:00	Donut or Danish Coffee	1 2 cups		1–2 starch 1–2 fat (2 CHO)
Lunch Noon	Sandwich Bread Lunch meat Chips Cookie Diet soda	 2 slices 4 slices 1 pkg (¾ oz) 1 large	With light mayo	4–5 starch 3–4 meat 2–3 fat (4–5 CHO)
Snack 3:00	Apple or cookie	1		1–2 starch 1–2 fat (2 CHO)
Dinner 6:30	Chicken/pork chop Potatoes/rice Roll or bread Vegetable or salad Milk, 2% Fruit	3–4 oz 1 cup 1 1 cup 1	Broiled With margarine With margarine With light dressing	3–4 meat 3 starch 1–2 vegetable 1 milk 1 fruit 2–3 fat (5–6 CHO)
Evening 10:30	Ice cream/cookies/fruit	1 cup		2–3 starch 1–2 fat (2 CHO)

300 g CHO (46%)
105 g protein (16%)
110 g fat (38%)
2600–2700 kcal

FIGURE 9A: Modified Food/Meal Plan Based on the Food History in Figure 8A

Name __Betty Jones__   Date __Jan 4__

	Bkfst 7:00–7:30	Snack	Lunch 12:00	Snack	Dinner 6:30	Snack 10:00	Total servings/day	CHO (g)	Protein (g)	Fat (g)	Kcal
Starch	1–2	0–1	2–3		2–3	1–2	10	15 / 150	3 / 30	1 / 10	80
Fruit	1		0–1	0–1	1		3	15 / 45			60
Milk	1 (1%)				1		2	12 / 24	8 / 16	1 / 4	90
Veg					1–2		2	5 / 10	2 / 4		25
Meat/Sub			2–3		3–4		5		7 / 35	5(3) / 25	75(55)
Fat	0–1	0–1	1–2	0–1	1–2	0–1	6			5 / 30	45
CHO choices	3–4	0–1	3–4	0–1	4–5	1–2	**Total grams**	229	85	69	**Total = 1800–1900**
							Kcal/gram	×4 / 916	×4 / 340	×9 / 621	
							Percent kcal	49%	18%	33%	

TABLE 4A: Human Insulin Preparations

Type of Insulin	Onset of Action	Peak Action	Usual Effective Duration	Monitor Effect After
Rapid acting Lispro Aspart	<15 min	0.5–1.5 h	2–4 h	2 h
Short acting Regular	0.5–1 h	2–3 h	3–6 h	4 h
Intermediate acting NPH Lente	2–4 h 3–4 h	6–10 h 6–12 h	10–16 h 12–18 h	8–12 h 8–12 h
Long acting Ultralente Glargine	6–10 h 1.1 h	10–16 h —	18–20 h 24 h	10–12 h 10–12 h
Mixtures 70/30 (70% NPH, 30% regular) 50/50 (50% NPH, 50% regular) 75/25 (75% neutral protamine lispro [NPL], 25% lispro)	0.5–1 h	Dual	10–16 h	

FIGURE 10A: Sample Documentation Form

Name _____ Date _____ Provider _____

Referred by _____ Age _____ Onset of diabetes _____

☐ Group ☐ Individual consult ☐ Initial visit ☐ Follow-up

Current diabetes medications: _____

		Assessment:								Food plan kcal		
Ht	Wt goal									g	CHO	PRO	FAT
Wt	Wt △									%			
			Breakfast	Snack	Lunch	Snack	Dinner	Snack		Intervention/education		
Exercise		Time								☐ nutrition goals		
Frequency										☐ meal spacing/timing		
Alcohol use		CHO Choices:								☐ portions/consistency ☐ CHO counting ☐ exchanges ☐ other		
		Starches/Fruits/Milk								☐ label reading		
A1C	Chol	Veg								☐ snack choices		
BG	LDL	Meat								☐ fat ☐ eating out		
BP	HDL	Fat								☐ alcohol ☐ sodium		
	TG									☐ hypoglycemia		
Meds		Comments/plan:								☐ sick day management ☐ intensification ☐ exercise ☐ other		
Complications										Level of complexity:		
										Times spent:		

Reprinted with permission from the International Diabetes Center, Minneapolis, MN.

About the American Diabetes Association

The American Diabetes Association is the nation's leading voluntary health organization supporting diabetes research, information, and advocacy. Its mission is to prevent and cure diabetes and to improve the lives of all people affected by diabetes. The American Diabetes Association is the leading publisher of comprehensive diabetes information. Its huge library of practical and authoritative books for people with diabetes covers every aspect of self-care—cooking and nutrition, fitness, weight control, medications, complications, emotional issues, and general self-care.

To order American Diabetes Association books: Call 1-800-232-6733. Or log on to http://store.diabetes.org

To join the American Diabetes Association: Call 1-800-806-7801. www.diabetes.org/membership

For more information about diabetes or ADA programs and services: Call 1-800-342-2383. E-mail: Customerservice@diabetes.org or log on to www.diabetes.org

To locate an ADA/NCQA Recognized Provider of quality diabetes care in your area: www.ncqa.org/dprp/

To find an ADA Recognized Education Program in your area: Call 1-888-232-0822. www.diabetes.org/recognition/education.asp

To join the fight to increase funding for diabetes research, end discrimination, and improve insurance coverage: Call 1-800-342-2383. www.diabetes.org/advocacy

To find out how you can get involved with the programs in your community: Call 1-800-342-2383. See below for program Web addresses.

- *American Diabetes Month:* Educational activities aimed at those diagnosed with diabetes—month of November. www.diabetes.org/ADM
- *American Diabetes Alert:* Annual public awareness campaign to find the undiagnosed—held the fourth Tuesday in March. www.diabetes.org/alert
- *The Diabetes Assistance & Resources Program (DAR):* diabetes awareness program targeted to the Latino community. www.diabetes.org/DAR
- *African American Program:* diabetes awareness program targeted to the African American community. www.diabetes.org/africanamerican
- *Awakening the Spirit: Pathways to Diabetes Prevention & Control:* diabetes awareness program targeted to the Native American community. www.diabetes.org/awakening

To find out about an important research project regarding type 2 diabetes: www.diabetes.org/ada/research.asp

To obtain information on making a planned gift or charitable bequest: Call 1-888-700-7029. www.diabetes.org/ada/plan.asp

To make a donation or memorial contribution: Call 1-800-342-2383. www.diabetes.org/ada/cont.asp